CARDIOVAS CULAR WELLNESS

A Comprehensive Guide

To A

Healthier Heart

Dr Buford L Brown

Table of contents

Introduction

Within the intricate symphony of life, an organ reigns supreme, orchestrating the very essence of our existence—the heart. A silent sentinel, it tirelessly pumps the elixir of life through the complex network of our veins and arteries, fueling our bodies with vitality and vigor. Often taken for granted, the heart is the true maestro of our well-being, its melody the life force of our existence.

But what lies beneath the rhythmic cadence of this remarkable organ is an entire universe of wonder—a realm where science and spirituality converge, where the secrets of longevity and vitality are unveiled. Welcome to the world of "Cardiovascular Wellness," a journey deep into the heart of our being that promises not only to captivate your mind but also to transform your life.

As we turn the pages that follow, we embark on an extraordinary voyage, guided by the latest scientific discoveries and ancient wisdom, to unravel the mysteries of the cardiovascular system and its profound impact on our overall well-being. We will traverse the labyrinthine corridors of arteries, delve into the intricate chemistry of blood, and explore the profound connection between our heart and soul.

Prepare to be awestruck by the elegance of the heart's design, the resilience of the cardiovascular system, and the astonishing potential it holds to enhance the quality of our lives. "Cardiovascular Wellness" is not just a book; it is a revelation, a testament to the intricate harmony of science and spirituality, and an invitation to embark on a transformative journey toward a healthier, more vibrant existence.

So, fasten your seatbelts, dear reader, for we are about to embark on an odyssey that will leave you spellbound, forever changing the way you perceive your heart, your health, and your life. Welcome to the epic tale of "Cardiovascular Wellness."

Book Description

Embark on an extraordinary journey to unlock the secrets of lasting vitality and well-being with "Cardiovascular Wellness." In a world filled with health-related uncertainties, this book stands as your beacon of hope, guiding you towards a healthier, more vibrant life. Here, we delve deep into the realm of heart health, answering burning questions that have lingered in your mind for too long.

Are you concerned about the state of your heart as you age? Worried about the ticking time bomb of heart disease and stroke?

"Cardiovascular Wellness" offers the answers you seek, demystifying the complexities of cardiovascular health. You will find not only solutions but also a newfound sense of empowerment, knowing that you hold the key to your well-being.

Let's explore why this book is your essential companion on the path to cardiovascular wellness:

The Roadmap to Heart Health: This book provides a comprehensive and meticulously crafted roadmap to bolster your cardiovascular health. Navigate the intricate network of your circulatory system with ease, armed with knowledge that can save lives.

Cutting-Edge Insights: Stay at the forefront of heart wellness with the latest research and expert insights. Unravel the mysteries of your heart's inner workings and discover how to optimise its function.

Practical Guidance: Say goodbye to the confusion surrounding heart-healthy lifestyle choices. "Cardiovascular Wellness" offers practical tips tailored to your unique needs, making it easier than ever to implement lasting changes.

Inspirational Stories: Meet individuals who have faced heart health challenges head-on and emerged victorious. Their stories will inspire you to take action and reclaim your vitality.

What can you expect as you dive into this enlightening journey?

Empowerment: Take charge of your heart health with newfound confidence. Say goodbye to anxiety and uncertainty, knowing that you are equipped with the tools to thrive.

Clarity: Finally, gain a comprehensive understanding of what truly works for your heart. No more sifting through conflicting advice – this book provides clarity and direction.

Energy: Experience a remarkable surge of energy and well-being as you implement the principles of cardiovascular wellness. Feel the rejuvenation of your body and spirit.

Longevity: Unleash your potential for a longer, healthier life. Live each day with the peace of mind that comes from knowing you are nurturing your most vital organ.

With "Cardiovascular Wellness," you're not just reading a book; you're embarking on a life-changing odyssey towards a future filled with boundless energy and enduring vitality. Say goodbye to doubt and hesitation; your transformation into a healthier, happier you awaits within these pages. Let the journey begin!

Chapter One

What is cardiovascular Disease

Cardiovascular disease (CVD) stands as a formidable adversary on the global health stage, a pervasive and insidious threat to human well-being that has transcended boundaries of age, gender, and geography. This chapter embarks on an elaborate journey into the intricate landscape of cardiovascular health, aiming to provide an impressive and comprehensive understanding of this multifaceted malady. Our quest is to equip readers with the knowledge and tools to attain cardiovascular wellness and lead fulfilling, heart-healthy lives.

I. Understanding Cardiovascular Disease:

The Prevalence of CVD:

1. Cardiovascular disease encompasses a class of conditions that afflict the heart and blood vessels. It stands as the leading cause of death worldwide, responsible for a significant proportion of global mortality.

The Spectrum of CVD:

2. CVD encompasses various disorders, including coronary artery disease (CAD), heart failure, stroke, hypertension, and peripheral artery disease (PAD). Each of these conditions exhibits unique characteristics and consequences.

II. Risk Factors and Causes:

Genetics and Family History:

Genetic predisposition plays a pivotal role in the development of CVD. Understanding one's familial history can provide valuable insights into susceptibilLifestyle Factors:

Lifestyle choices significantly impact cardiovascular health. Poor dietary habits, sedentary lifestyles, smoking, and excessive alcohol consumption are prominent risk factors.

Metabolic Factors:

Conditions such as diabetes and obesity contribute substantially to CVD risk. They affect the body's metabolic processes and increase the likelihood of vascular complications.

III. Pathophysiology and Mechanisms:

Atherosclerosis:

The hallmark of CVD is atherosclerosis, a complex process involving the gradual accumulation of plaque within arterial walls. This process narrows the arteries, reducing blood flow and causing ischemic events.

Inflammation and Oxidative Stress:

Chronic inflammation and oxidative stress exacerbate CVD by damaging vascular tissues and promoting plaque formation.

Hypertension:

Elevated blood pressure strains the cardiovascular system, increasing the risk of heart disease, stroke, and other complications.

IV. Diagnostic Tools and Imaging:

Non-Invasive Tests:

Advanced diagnostic tools such as echocardiography, electrocardiography (ECG), and stress tests help clinicians assess cardiac function without invasive procedures.

Imaging Modalities:

Cutting-edge imaging technologies like cardiac MRI and CT angiography offer precise visualization of cardiac structures and blood vessels, aiding in diagnosis and treatment planning.

V. Prevention and Management:

Lifestyle Modifications:

Achieving cardiovascular wellness necessitates lifestyle changes, including a heart-healthy diet, regular exercise, smoking cessation, and moderation in alcohol consumption.

Medications:

Pharmacological interventions can control blood pressure, lower cholesterol levels, and manage diabetes, reducing the risk of CVD complications.

Surgical and Interventional Procedures:

In severe cases, surgical interventions such as angioplasty, stent placement, or coronary artery bypass grafting (CABG) may be necessary to restore blood flow to the heart.

VI. Emerging Research and Innovations:

Precision Medicine:

1. Advancements in genetic and molecular research are paving the way for personalized approaches to CVD prevention and treatment.

Stem Cell Therapy:

2. Cutting-edge therapies, including stem cell treatments, hold promise in regenerating damaged heart tissues and improving cardiac function.

Chapter Two

Introduction: Maintaining a healthy heart

In the intricate tapestry of human existence, few threads are as crucial as the beating rhythm of our hearts. The heart, that resilient muscle nestled within the protective confines of our ribcage, is the life force that sustains us from the very moment we take our first breath to the last sigh we breathe. It is the symphony conductor of our body's orchestra, orchestrating the circulation of life-giving blood that fuels every cell, every tissue, and every organ. Its significance to our overall well-being is immeasurable, for the state of our heart is tantamount to the state of our existence.

Welcome to the illuminating journey that is "Cardiovascular Wellness." This comprehensive volume is a testament to the profound importance of maintaining a healthy heart in the pursuit of a long, vibrant, and fulfilling life. Within these pages, we will embark on a voyage of discovery, uncovering the intricacies of cardiovascular health, and unraveling the myriad factors that impact the well-being of this vital organ.

In this meticulously crafted book, we will delve deep into the realm of cardiovascular wellness, exploring not only the anatomy and physiology of the heart but also the intricate web of lifestyle choices, genetic predispositions, and environmental influences that can either fortify or jeopardize our cardiac health. We will navigate through the maze of heart-healthy diets, exercise regimens, and stress management techniques, all while shedding light on the latest advancements in medical science and technology that hold the promise of extending the longevity and vitality of our most precious organ.

The pages that follow are a treasure trove of knowledge, carefully curated to empower you with the insights and tools necessary to embark on your own journey toward cardiovascular wellness. Whether you are a healthcare professional seeking to expand your expertise, a concerned individual eager to safeguard their heart, or simply a curious soul thirsty for knowledge, "Cardiovascular Wellness" invites you to explore the boundless possibilities that arise when one takes control of their heart health.

So, join us as we embark on this enlightening expedition into the heart of cardiovascular wellness, where every chapter, every paragraph, and every word is a testament to the profound significance of nurturing the heart—a journey that promises to not only elongate the years of your life but, more importantly, enhance the quality of each heartbeat.

Chapter Three

The Anatomy of the Heart

The Heart's Role in Cardiovascular Wellness

To appreciate the significance of heart disease and its risk factors, one must first grasp the intricate anatomy of the heart. The heart, a muscular organ the size of a clenched fist, consists of four chambers: two atria and two ventricles. These chambers work in perfect harmony to facilitate the circulation of blood, which carries vital nutrients and oxygen to the body's tissues

Types of Heart Disease

Exploring the Spectrum

There is no one-size-fits-all when it comes to heart disease. It manifests in various forms, each with its own unique characteristics and risk factors. We will discuss conditions such as coronary artery disease (CAD), heart failure, arrhythmias, and congenital heart defects, providing insights into their causes, symptoms, and potential outcomes.

Risk Factors for Heart Disease

The Culprits Behind Cardiovascular Concerns

Understanding heart disease requires a keen awareness of the risk factors that contribute to its development. These factors can be categorised into two main types: modifiable and non-modifiable.

Modifiable risk factors include lifestyle choices such as diet, physical activity, and smoking, while non-modifiable factors encompass genetics, age, and gender.

Modifiable Risk Factors

Taking Charge of Your Heart Health

This chapter delves into modifiable risk factors in depth, offering guidance on how individuals can take proactive steps to mitigate their risk. Strategies for adopting a heart-healthy diet, engaging in regular exercise, and quitting smoking are discussed, along with the profound impact these lifestyle changes can have on cardiovascular wellness.

Non-Modifiable Risk Factors

The Hand You're Dealt

While some risk factors are beyond our control, it is essential to understand how genetics, age, and gender influence heart disease risk. We explore the latest research on genetic predispositions, the effects of aging on the heart, and the unique considerations for men and women regarding cardiovascular health.

Emerging Risk Factors

The Evolving Landscape of Heart Disease

As science advances, so does our understanding of heart disease. This chapter explores emerging risk factors, including the role of inflammation, stress, sleep, and air pollution in cardiovascular health. These insights provide a glimpse into the ever-evolving field of cardiology and the potential avenues for future prevention and treatment.

Diagnosis and Screening

The Path to Early Detection

Early detection of heart disease is crucial for effective management. This chapter outlines the various diagnostic tools and screening tests available, from electrocardiograms (ECGs) to advanced imaging techniques. We also discuss the importance of routine check-ups and when to seek medical attention for concerning symptoms.

Treatment and Management

Improving Cardiovascular Outcomes

When heart disease strikes, timely and appropriate treatment is paramount. In this chapter, we explore the diverse array of treatment options, including medications, lifestyle interventions, and surgical procedures. Moreover, we delve into the concept of multidisciplinary care, emphasizing the role of healthcare providers in guiding patients toward cardiovascular wellness.

Preventing Heart Disease

Empowering a Heart-Healthy Future

We conclude our journey with a comprehensive discussion on prevention strategies. By combining knowledge of risk factors, healthy lifestyle choices, early detection, and access to quality healthcare, individuals can proactively reduce their risk of heart disease and promote their own cardiovascular wellness.

Conclusion

In "Cardiovascular Wellness," we have embarked on an extensive exploration of heart disease and its risk factors. With knowledge as our guide, we empower readers to take control of their heart health, promoting not only longevity but also a higher quality of life. As we close this chapter, remember that the journey to cardiovascular wellness is a lifelong endeavor—one that each of us can embark upon, one heartbeat at a time.

Chapter Four

Exercise

The human heart is a remarkable organ, tirelessly pumping blood throughout our bodies, ensuring the delivery of oxygen and nutrients to every cell. To build and maintain a healthy heart, it's crucial to engage in regular exercise. This not only strengthens the heart muscle but also enhances its efficiency, lowers the risk of cardiovascular diseases, and improves overall well-being. In this comprehensive guide, we will explore various exercises that are specifically designed to build and fortify the heart.

Aerobic Exercise:

1. Aerobic exercises, also known as cardiovascular exercises, are paramount in heart health. These activities increase your heart rate and breathing, training the heart to work more efficiently. Some popular aerobic exercises include:

   - Running: This high-intensity exercise not only strengthens the heart but also burns calories.
   - Cycling: A low-impact exercise that provides an excellent cardiovascular workout.
   - Swimming: Engaging in laps in the pool is gentle on the joints and highly effective for heart health.

Interval Training:

Interval training involves alternating between short bursts of high-intensity exercise and brief periods of rest or lower-intensity activity. This approach challenges the heart to adapt quickly and can lead to significant improvements in cardiovascular fitness.

Strength Training:

While cardiovascular exercises are essential, don't overlook the importance of strength training. Building muscle can help improve metabolism and overall cardiovascular health. Incorporate exercises like:

Weightlifting: Focusing on compound movements like squats, deadlifts, and bench presses.

Resistance Bands: These versatile tools can be used for resistance exercises that target various muscle groups.

Yoga and Tai Chi:

These mind-body practices emphasize deep breathing, relaxation, and gentle movements. While not as intense as some other exercises, they promote relaxation and reduce stress, which is beneficial for heart health.

Hiking and Nature Walks:

Enjoying the great outdoors through activities like hiking and walking in nature not only gets your heart rate up but also provides the added benefit of stress reduction.

Dancing:

Dancing is a fun way to get your heart pumping. Whether it's ballroom, hip-hop, or salsa, dancing offers a great cardiovascular workout.

High-Intensity Interval Training (HIIT):

HIIT workouts involve short, intense bursts of exercise followed by brief rest periods. This approach can significantly boost heart health in a shorter amount of time compared to traditional workouts.

Circuit Training:

Circuit training combines strength and aerobic exercises in a structured routine. Moving from one exercise to another with minimal rest keeps the heart rate elevated.

CrossFit:

CrossFit is a high-intensity fitness program that incorporates a variety of exercises, including weightlifting, running, and bodyweight movements, to improve overall fitness and heart health.

Swimming:

Swimming is a full-body workout that is gentle on the joints, making it suitable for people of all ages. It improves heart health by increasing endurance and strengthening the cardiovascular system.

Incorporating a variety of these exercises into your fitness routine can help you build and maintain a strong and healthy heart. Remember to consult with a healthcare professional before starting any new exercise program, especially if you have pre existing medical conditions or concerns about your heart health. Listen to your body, stay consistent, and reap the benefits of a strong and resilient heart.

Foods that are beneficial to the heart

A heart-healthy diet is crucial for maintaining cardiovascular health and reducing the risk of heart disease. Let's explore an impressive list of foods that are beneficial to the heart:

Oily Fish: Salmon, mackerel, and trout are rich in omega-3 fatty acids, which can help lower blood pressure and reduce the risk of heart disease.

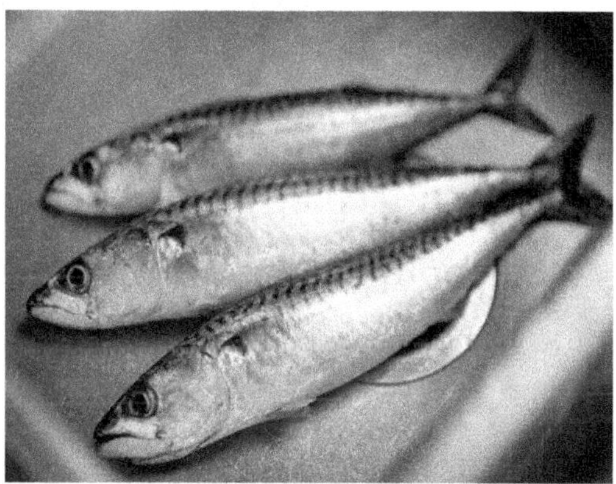

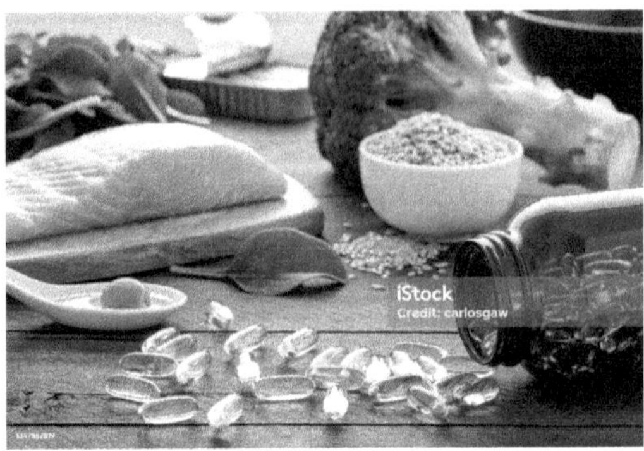

Berries: Blueberries, strawberries, and raspberries are packed with antioxidants that can help reduce inflammation and improve heart health.

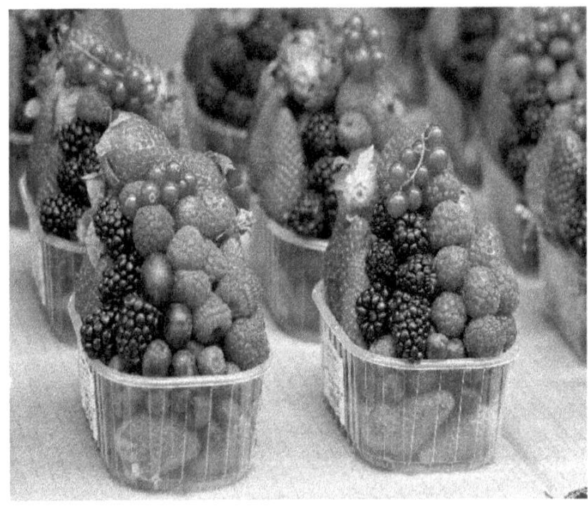

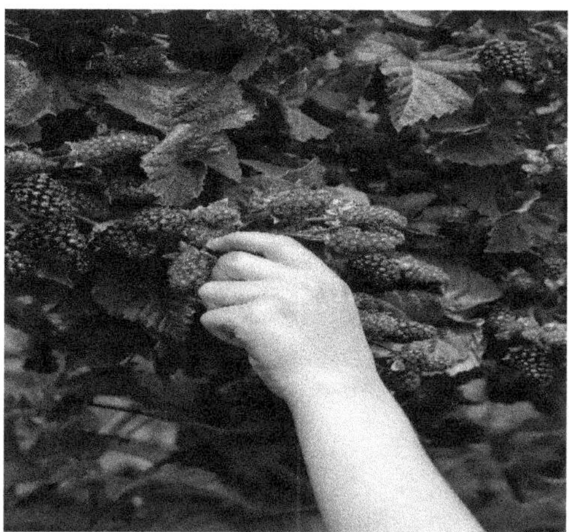

3. Nuts: Almonds, walnuts, and pistachios contain healthy fats, fibre, and antioxidants that support heart health.

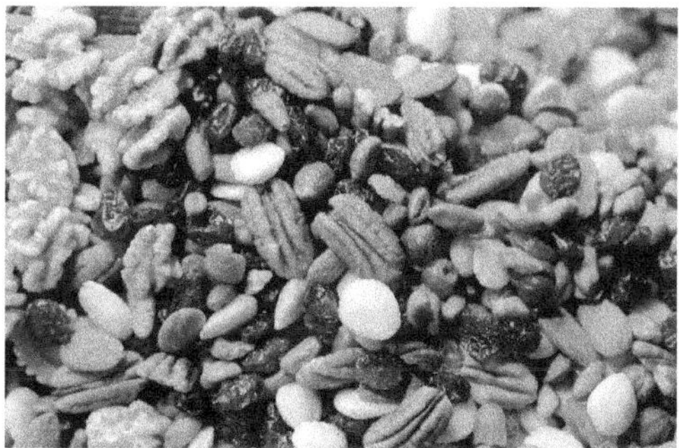

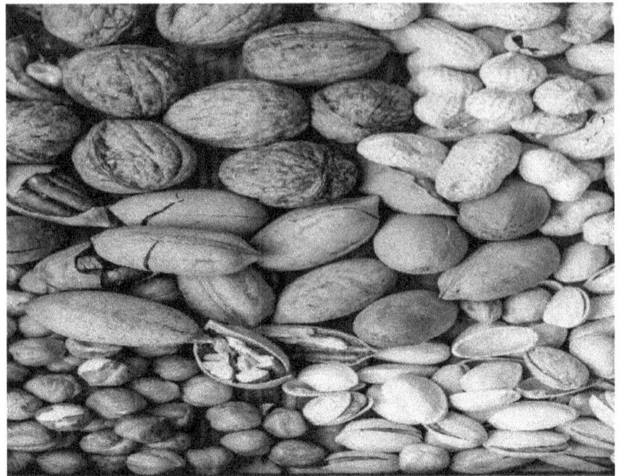

Oats: High in soluble fiber, oats can help lower cholesterol levels and improve heart health.

Leafy Greens: Spinach, kale, and Swiss chard are loaded with vitamins, minerals, and antioxidants that promote heart health.

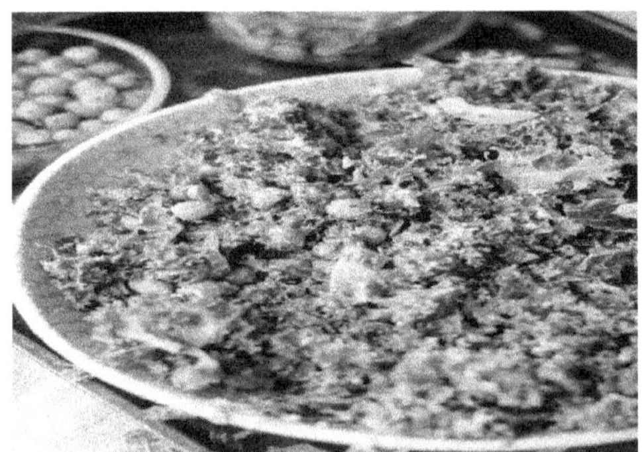

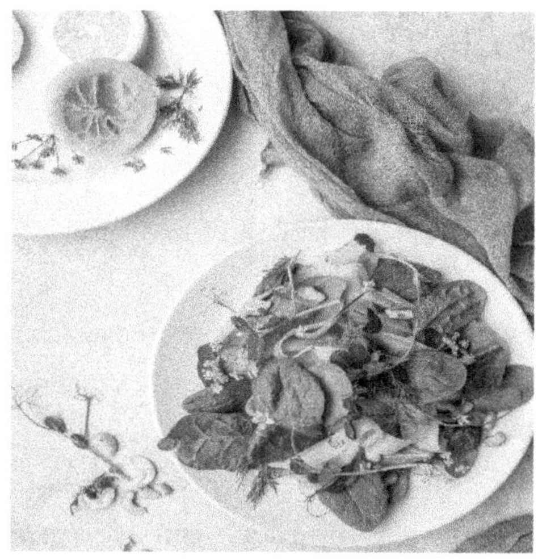

Avocado: Rich in monounsaturated fats, avocados can help lower bad cholesterol levels and reduce the risk of heart disease.

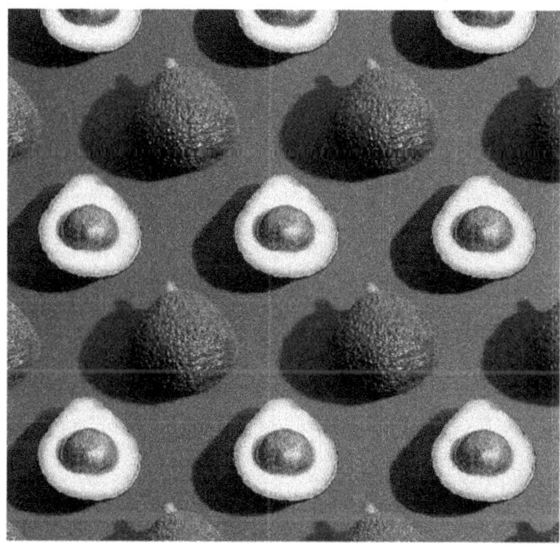

7. Legumes: Beans, lentils, and chickpeas are excellent sources of plant-based protein and fiber, which can benefit heart health.

8. Olive Oil: Extra virgin olive oil is a healthy source of monounsaturated fats and antioxidants that support heart health.

9. Dark Chocolate: In moderation, dark chocolate (70% cocoa or higher) may improve heart health due to its flavonoid content.

10. Tomatoes: These are packed with lycopene, which has been linked to a reduced risk of heart disease.

11. Garlic: Garlic contains allicin, which may help lower blood pressure and reduce the risk of heart disease.

12. Flaxseeds: These tiny seeds are rich in omega-3 fatty acids, fiber, and lignans, all of which support heart health.

13. Green Tea: The antioxidants in green tea, like catechins, may help lower cholesterol levels and reduce the risk of heart disease.

14. Whole Grains: Foods like brown rice, quinoa, and whole wheat bread are rich in fiber and nutrients that promote heart health.

15. Pomegranates: Packed with antioxidants, pomegranates may help improve cholesterol levels and reduce blood pressure.

16. Red Wine: In moderation, red wine contains resveratrol, which may have heart-protective effects.

Fatty Fish: Besides omega-3s, fish like sardines and herring are also high in vitamin D, which is beneficial for heart health.

Turmeric: This spice contains curcumin, which has anti-inflammatory and antioxidant properties that may benefit the heart.

Walnuts: These nuts are a good source of alpha-linolenic acid (ALA), another type of omega-3 fatty acid.

Oranges: Citrus fruits like oranges are rich in vitamin C and fiber, which can support heart health.

Remember that a heart-healthy diet should be part of an overall healthy lifestyle that includes regular exercise, maintaining a healthy weight, and avoiding smoking. Incorporating these foods into your diet can contribute to a strong and healthy heart.

Chapter Six

Experimental analysis and health check

In an era where data-driven decisions and preventive healthcare are paramount, conducting an experimental analysis and health check has become indispensable. This comprehensive process employs cutting-edge technologies and methodologies to assess an individual's physical, mental, and emotional well-being. This impressive endeavor seeks to provide a holistic understanding of one's health status, enabling tailored interventions for a healthier and happier life.

Methodology:

Advanced Diagnostics: Our analysis commences with state-of-the-art diagnostic tools. From 3D body scans to DNA profiling, we delve deep into the individual's biological makeup, uncovering hidden health markers.

Biometric Monitoring: Continuous monitoring of vital signs, including heart rate, blood pressure, and sleep patterns, allows for real-time health assessment. Wearable technology and smart sensors ensure precise data collection.

Metabolomics and Microbiome Analysis: Exploring the metabolic profile and gut microbiome composition unveils insights into nutrient absorption, metabolism, and overall gut health. This advanced analysis guides dietary recommendations.

4. Psychological Assessment: Mental health is a crucial aspect of well-being. Psychological assessments, including personality profiling and emotional intelligence evaluation, are performed by experts to provide a holistic view of an individual's emotional state.

5. Environmental Impact: Analyzing an individual's living environment for pollutants, allergens, and other potential health hazards is integral to this process. Indoor air quality, water purity, and ergonomic assessments are carried out.

6. Artificial Intelligence Integration: Advanced AI algorithms process the vast amount of data collected, identifying patterns, trends, and potential health risks. Machine learning models predict future health outcomes and suggest personalized wellness strategies.

Benefits:

1. Early Disease Detection: Our experimental analysis can identify health issues at their earliest stages, facilitating timely intervention and potentially saving lives.

2. Personalized Health Plans: Based on the extensive data gathered, personalized health plans are developed. These encompass tailored nutrition, fitness routines, and mental well-being strategies.

3. Improved Quality of Life: By addressing underlying health factors and providing guidance for lifestyle modifications, individuals can experience enhanced energy levels, mental clarity, and overall happiness.

4. Data-Driven Decision-Making: The wealth of data generated empowers individuals to make informed decisions about their health and well-being. It serves as a valuable resource for healthcare providers as well.

5. Cost Savings: Prevention is more cost-effective than treatment. Identifying and addressing health concerns early can significantly reduce healthcare expenditu

Chapter Seven

Creating a Heart Health Plan for the Future

Creating a comprehensive and forward-thinking Heart Health Plan is essential for ensuring a long and healthy life. In today's fast-paced world, where sedentary lifestyles and unhealthy dietary choices have become the norm, it's more critical than ever to lay the foundation for a heart-healthy future. This plan will encompass various aspects of your life, from nutrition and exercise to stress management and regular medical check-ups, all designed to promote optimal cardiovascular well-being.

Nutrition:

A well-balanced and heart-healthy diet is the cornerstone of any plan for cardiovascular health. Your future Heart Health Plan should include:

1. Fruits and Vegetables: Aim to consume a variety of colorful fruits and vegetables rich in antioxidants and fiber. These can help reduce the risk of heart disease by lowering cholesterol levels and supporting overall heart health.

2. Lean Proteins: Incorporate lean sources of protein, such as poultry, fish, beans, and tofu, into your meals. Limit

red meat and processed meats, as they are associated with an increased risk of heart disease.

Whole Grains: Choose whole grains like oats, quinoa, and whole wheat over refined grains. They provide essential nutrients and fiber that can help lower your risk of heart disease.

Healthy Fats: Opt for unsaturated fats found in olive oil, avocados, and nuts. These fats can help improve your cholesterol profile and reduce inflammation in your arteries.

Limit Sodium: Reduce your sodium intake by avoiding highly processed foods and excessive salt. High sodium intake can lead to high blood pressure, a major risk factor for heart diseas

Exercise:

Regular physical activity is crucial for maintaining heart health. Your plan should include:

Cardiovascular Exercise: Aim for at least 150 minutes of moderate-intensity aerobic exercise or 75 minutes of vigorous-intensity exercise per week. Activities like brisk walking, jogging, cycling, or swimming can strengthen your heart and improve circulation.

Strength Training: Incorporate strength training exercises at least two days a week to build muscle mass, boost metabolism, and improve overall fitness.

3. Flexibility and Balance: Don't forget about flexibility and balance exercises, which can help reduce the risk of falls and injuries as you age.

Stress Management:

Chronic stress can negatively impact your heart health. Your Heart Health Plan should include strategies to manage stress, such as:

1. Mindfulness and Meditation: Practice mindfulness techniques and meditation to reduce stress and promote emotional well-being.

2. Relaxation Techniques: Explore relaxation techniques like deep breathing, progressive muscle relaxation, or yoga to calm your mind and body.

3. Time Management: Efficiently manage your time to reduce the stress associated with a hectic lifestyle.

Regular Check-ups:

Scheduled medical check-ups are essential for early detection and prevention of heart-related issues. Your plan should include:

1. Annual Physicals: Visit your healthcare provider for an annual physical examination, including blood pressure, cholesterol, and blood sugar checks.

2. Screenings: Follow recommended screenings for heart disease risk factors, such as lipid profiles, electrocardiograms (ECGs), and stress tests as needed.

3. Medication Management: If prescribed medication, take it as directed and attend regular medication reviews with your healthcare provider.

4. Lifestyle Assessments: Periodically reassess your lifestyle choices and adapt your Heart Health Plan as needed.

Social Connections:

Maintaining healthy relationships and social connections can positively impact your heart health. Incorporate activities and practices that promote social well-being into your plan.

Family and Friends: Spend quality time with loved ones and engage in activities that foster connections and emotional support.

Community Involvement: Participate in community groups or volunteer work to build a sense of purpose and belonging.

Sleep:

Adequate sleep is crucial for heart health. Aim for 7-9 hours of quality sleep per night to support overall well-being.

Addiction

Addiction is a widespread and pressing issue in today's society, affecting millions of individuals worldwide. While it is commonly associated with its detrimental impact on mental health, it is essential to recognize that addiction can also have severe consequences for physical health, particularly when it comes to cardiovascular disease. This complex relationship between addiction and cardiovascular health underscores the need for effective interventions, and one such resource that offers valuable insights is the book titled "Cardiovascular Wellness."

Cardiovascular disease, encompassing conditions such as hypertension, coronary artery disease, and stroke, ranks as the leading cause of death globally. It is well-documented that addiction, whether to substances like nicotine, alcohol, or illicit drugs, or behavioral addictions like gambling, can significantly exacerbate the risk and severity of cardiovascular disease. Understanding the mechanisms behind this relationship is crucial for both healthcare providers and individuals struggling with addiction.

Firstly, substances like tobacco and alcohol, when abused, can directly harm the cardiovascular system. Nicotine, found in cigarettes, raises blood pressure and heart rate, constricts blood vessels, and damages the lining of arteries – all of which increase the likelihood of heart disease. Similarly, excessive alcohol consumption can lead to high blood pressure, cardiomyopathy (weakening of the heart muscle), and irregular heart rhythms.

Secondly, addiction often goes hand-in-hand with unhealthy lifestyle choices. Individuals grappling with addiction may neglect proper nutrition, exercise, and sleep, all of which are essential components of cardiovascular wellness. This neglect can contribute to weight gain, diabetes, and elevated cholesterol levels, further elevating the risk of heart disease.

Furthermore, the stress and anxiety associated with addiction can stimulate the release of stress hormones like cortisol, which, when chronically elevated, can damage the cardiovascular system. Additionally, addiction can lead to social isolation and strained relationships, which can exacerbate stress and negatively impact mental health, further influencing cardiovascular health.

So, how can the book "Cardiovascular Wellness" make a difference in the lives of individuals battling addiction and struggling with cardiovascular health issues? This book serves as a comprehensive guide to understanding and improving heart health, offering practical advice and strategies that can benefit anyone, but especially those dealing with addiction-related challenges.

1. Education and Awareness: "Cardiovascular Wellness" provides clear, easily accessible information about cardiovascular health and the risks associated with addiction. It empowers readers with knowledge about the consequences of their actions, helping them make informed decisions.

2. Behavioral Change: The book emphasizes the importance of lifestyle changes, such as adopting a heart-healthy diet, engaging in regular physical activity, and managing stress. For individuals in recovery from addiction, these positive habits can replace harmful ones and improve overall well-being.

3. Emotional Well-being: "Cardiovascular Wellness" recognizes the emotional toll addiction can take and offers guidance on managing stress, anxiety, and depression. By addressing the psychological aspects of addiction, it provides valuable tools for mental and emotional healing.

4. Support and Motivation: The book includes personal stories of individuals who have successfully overcome addiction and improved their cardiovascular health. These inspiring narratives offer hope and motivation to readers who may be facing similar challenges.

5. Medical Insights: "Cardiovascular Wellness" also delves into the medical aspects of heart health, explaining the importance of regular check-ups, medication management, and working closely with healthcare

providers. This information is vital for individuals with a history of substance abuse, as they may require specialized care.

Chapter Nine

Maintenance of heart health

Maintaining heart health is of paramount importance, as the heart serves as the engine that powers the entire human body. A well-maintained heart not only ensures a longer and more fulfilling life but also reduces the risk of cardiovascular diseases, which remain a leading cause of mortality worldwide. In this comprehensive guide, we will delve into the multifaceted aspects of heart health maintenance, encompassing lifestyle choices, dietary habits, exercise routines, stress management, and medical interventions.

1. Dietary Habits:

    - A heart-healthy diet is a cornerstone of maintaining cardiac wellness. Focus on consuming a variety of nutrient-dense foods, including fruits, vegetables, whole grains, lean proteins, and healthy fats.
    - Reduce the intake of saturated and trans fats, which can elevate cholesterol levels and increase the risk of heart disease.
    - Limit sodium intake to control blood pressure and reduce the risk of hypertension.
    - Consume omega-3 fatty acids found in fatty fish like salmon, walnuts, and flaxseeds, as they can

help lower the risk of arrhythmias and atherosclerosis.

Stay hydrated and limit sugary beverages

Physical Activity:

Regular exercise is vital for heart health. Aim for at least 150 minutes of moderate-intensity aerobic activity or 75 minutes of vigorous-intensity aerobic activity each week.

Incorporate strength training exercises to build muscle mass and improve overall fitness.

Exercise improves circulation, reduces inflammation, and helps maintain a healthy weight, all of which contribute to heart health.

Stress Management:

Chronic stress can adversely affect the heart. Engage in stress-reduction techniques such as meditation, deep breathing exercises, yoga, or mindfulness to promote relaxation.

Maintain a healthy work-life balance to minimize stressors.

Smoking Cessation:

Smoking is a major risk factor for heart disease. Seek support to quit smoking and reduce your risk of heart-related problems.

Alcohol Moderation:

Limit alcohol consumption to moderate levels, as excessive drinking can contribute to high blood pressure and heart disease.

Regular Check-Ups:

Schedule regular check-ups with your healthcare provider. Monitoring blood pressure, cholesterol levels, and other cardiovascular risk factors is crucial.

Discuss family history of heart disease and consider genetic testing if necessary.

Medications and Medical Interventions:

If prescribed by a healthcare professional, take medications as directed to manage conditions such as high blood pressure, high cholesterol, or diabetes.

In some cases, medical interventions like angioplasty or coronary artery bypass surgery may be necessary to treat advanced heart disease.

Awareness and Education:

Stay informed about heart health through reputable sources, as knowledge empowers individuals to make informed decisions.

Learn to recognize the signs of a heart attack or stroke and seek immediate medical attention if they occur.

Support Systems:

Surround yourself with a supportive network of family and friends who encourage and enable your heart-healthy lifestyle choices.

Customised Approach:

Remember that everyone's heart health needs are unique. Consult with a healthcare provider to develop a personalized plan based on your specific risk factors and medical history.

The Heart

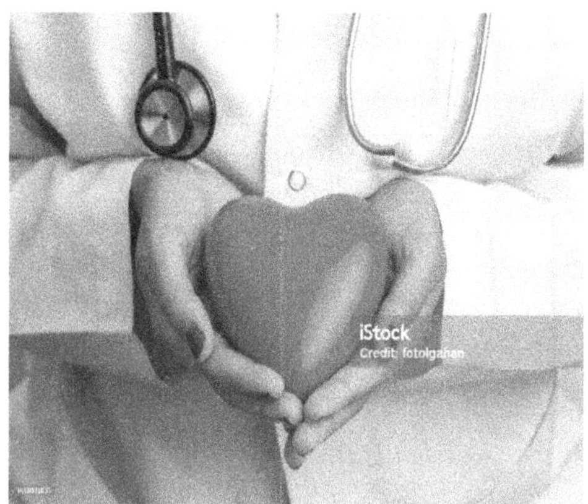

The human heart, an intricate and awe-inspiring organ, is often regarded as the symbol of life itself. Nestled within the protective confines of our ribcage, the heart tirelessly pumps blood, ensuring the delivery of oxygen and nutrients to every cell in our body. Its rhythmic beat is the soundtrack of our existence, a constant reminder of our vitality. In this essay, we will embark on a journey to explore the importance of cardiovascular wellness, focusing on the heart as its epicenter, and how maintaining its health can lead to a better life.

The Heart: Anatomy and Function

Before delving into the significance of cardiovascular wellness, it is crucial to understand the heart's anatomy and function. The heart is a muscular organ, roughly the size of a clenched fist, located slightly to the left of the chest's center. It consists of four chambers: two atria and two ventricles, each with a specific role in the circulatory system.

The right atrium receives deoxygenated blood from the body through the superior and inferior vena cava. It then contracts, sending this blood into the right ventricle. From there, the right ventricle pumps the blood into the pulmonary arteries, which transport it to the lungs for oxygenation. Oxygen-rich blood returns to the heart, entering the left atrium and then the left ventricle, which is responsible for pumping it out to nourish the entire body. This intricate sequence of events ensures a continuous flow of oxygen and nutrients to our tissues and organs.

Importance of Cardiovascular Wellness

Cardiovascular wellness, also known as heart health, encompasses a range of practices and habits that contribute to the well-being of the heart and the entire circulatory system. It is imperative to understand the importance of cardiovascular wellness, as it is intricately linked to our overall quality of life.

- Longevity: A healthy heart is synonymous with a longer life. By maintaining proper cardiovascular health, individuals are more likely to avoid heart-related diseases and complications, allowing them to enjoy a fuller, more extended life.

- Energy and Vitality: The heart pumps oxygen-rich blood to muscles and organs, providing the energy necessary for physical activities and daily tasks. A strong, efficient heart ensures that our body functions optimally, leading to increased vitality and improved endurance.

Reduced Risk of Disease: Cardiovascular wellness significantly reduces the risk of developing heart diseases such as coronary artery disease, heart attacks, and strokes. It also contributes to lower blood pressure, healthier cholesterol levels, and better blood sugar control.

Mental Wellbeing: The link between cardiovascular wellness and mental health is undeniable. Regular exercise, a cornerstone of heart health, releases endorphins, reducing stress and anxiety levels. A healthy heart can contribute to enhanced cognitive function and a reduced risk of conditions like dementia.

Quality of Life: A well-maintained cardiovascular system enhances one's overall quality of life. It allows individuals to partake in physical activities, travel, and enjoy life's pleasures without being limited by health concerns.

Achieving Cardiovascular Wellness

Now that we understand the significance of cardiovascular wellness, it's essential to explore how we can take steps to maintain a healthy heart and improve our overall well-being:

Regular Exercise: Engaging in regular physical activity, such as walking, jogging, swimming, or cycling, strengthens the heart muscle, improves circulation, and helps maintain a healthy weight.

2. Balanced Diet: Consuming a diet rich in fruits, vegetables, whole grains, lean proteins, and healthy fats supports heart health. Limiting processed foods, sodium, and sugar is crucial in preventing heart disease.

3. Stress Management: Chronic stress can have a detrimental impact on heart health. Practicing stress-reduction techniques like meditation, yoga, or deep breathing exercises can help maintain a healthy heart.

4. Regular Check-ups: Routine medical check-ups are essential to monitor blood pressure, cholesterol levels, and other risk factors. Early detection and management of issues can prevent more severe cardiovascular problems.

5. Avoiding Smoking and Excessive Alcohol: Smoking damages blood vessels and increases the risk of heart disease, while excessive alcohol consumption can lead to hypertension and heart failure. Quitting smoking and moderating alcohol intake is vital.

The heart is not only a vital organ but also a symbol of life's essence. The importance of cardiovascular wellness cannot be overstated, as it directly impacts our longevity, energy, and overall quality of life. By understanding the intricate workings of the heart and adopting heart-healthy practices, we can pave the way for a healthier and happier existence. Remember, the heart is not just an organ—it's the conductor of life's symphony, and taking care of it is our responsibility for a better, longer, and more fulfilling life.

Conclusion

In conclusion, "Cardiovascular Wellness: A Journey to Lifelong Health" serves as a comprehensive and enlightening exploration into the critical realm of heart health. Throughout the pages of this illuminating tome, we have delved deep into the intricacies of the cardiovascular system, dissected the myriad factors that impact our heart's well-being, and embarked on a transformative journey towards a lifetime of vitality.

This book has expertly unraveled the mysteries of cardiovascular health, providing a wealth of knowledge that empowers readers to take control of their own well-being. We have learned that a harmonious symphony of factors, from diet and exercise to stress management and genetics, orchestrates the fate of our hearts. With every turn of the page, we have gained invaluable insights into the power of prevention, the promise of early intervention, and the potential for remarkable rejuvenation.

As we conclude this journey, we are left with a profound appreciation for the incredible resilience and adaptability of the human heart. It is a reminder that our hearts, like the narrative within these pages, can be shaped and sculpted to withstand the tests of time. "Cardiovascular Wellness" is not merely a book but a call to action, an invitation to embrace a life imbued with vitality, and a testament to the enduring strength of the human spirit.

In the grand tapestry of our lives, the pursuit of cardiovascular wellness stands as a central thread, woven with knowledge, dedication, and a deep commitment to our own health. May this book serve as an enduring beacon of hope, a wellspring of wisdom, and a catalyst for transformation on the path to a heart-healthy and fulfilling life. Let it inspire us all to prioritize the well-being of our most vital organ, for in doing so, we unlock the potential for a future graced with boundless energy, lasting joy, and an abundance of heart.